INTRODUCTION

Reactor license renewal is an important part of the U.S. Nuclear Regulatory Commission's (NRC) mission to regulate the civilian use of nuclear materials to ensure adequate protection of public health and safety, to promote the common defense and security, and to protect the environment.

For the past 20 years, the NRC has been studying and refining the license renewal process. As of 2008, the NRC has renewed licenses for 26 facilities, which include 48 nuclear power reactors. Over the next 10 years, a large number of the remaining U.S. nuclear power facilities are expected to apply for 20-year operating license extensions.

This brochure provides information on the license renewal process, including the technical issues that nuclear plant owners consider before submitting an application and the criteria the NRC uses to evaluate a renewal request. This brochure will also introduce you to some of the NRC's highly skilled and uniquely qualified license renewal staff.

Additional information about the NRC can be found on the NRC's Web site (www.nrc.gov).

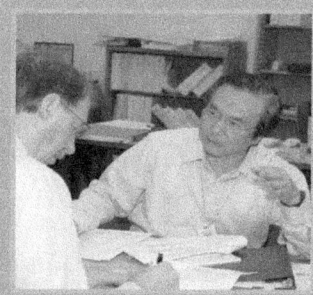

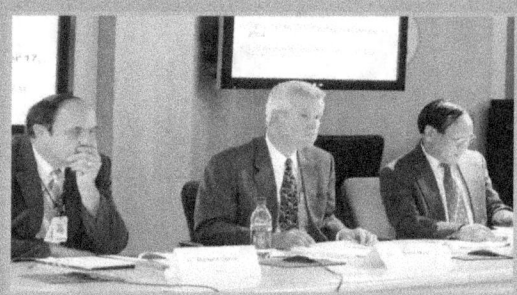

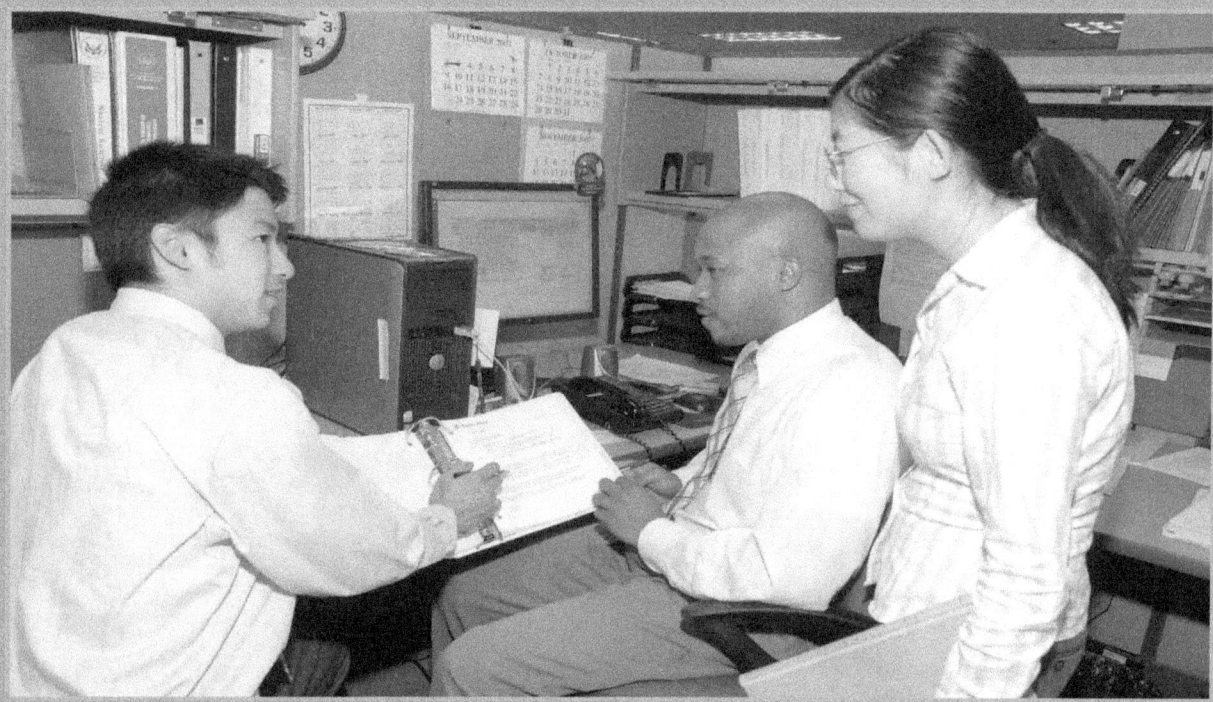

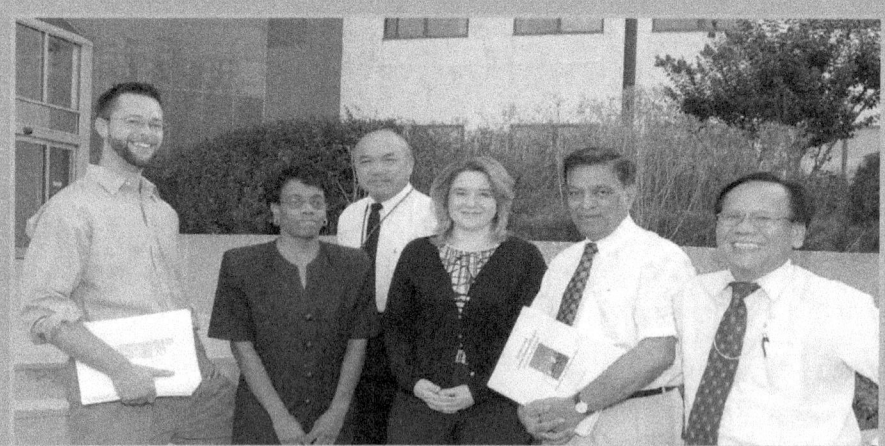

WHAT IS REACTOR LICENSE RENEWAL?

The NRC licenses and monitors all commercial nuclear power reactors operating in the United States. The initial licenses permit nuclear power reactors to operate for up to 40 years. After the initial period of operation, the NRC may grant a 20-year renewal of the operating license as long as the nuclear power facility owner can demonstrate that the facility will continue to operate safely for the extended period of operation.

NRC resident inspectors, who are stationed at each nuclear power facility, inspect and monitor nuclear power facilities daily for operational safety. Regional inspectors also conduct inspections throughout the year. The license renewal process, on the other hand, ensures that the plant can safely operate, with acceptable environmental impacts, during the period of extended operation.

Today nuclear energy provides about 20% of the electricity supply in the United States. The U.S. Energy Information Administration projects that total electricity demand will grow by 1.3% per year in the commercial sector and 2% in the residential sector from 2005 to 2030.

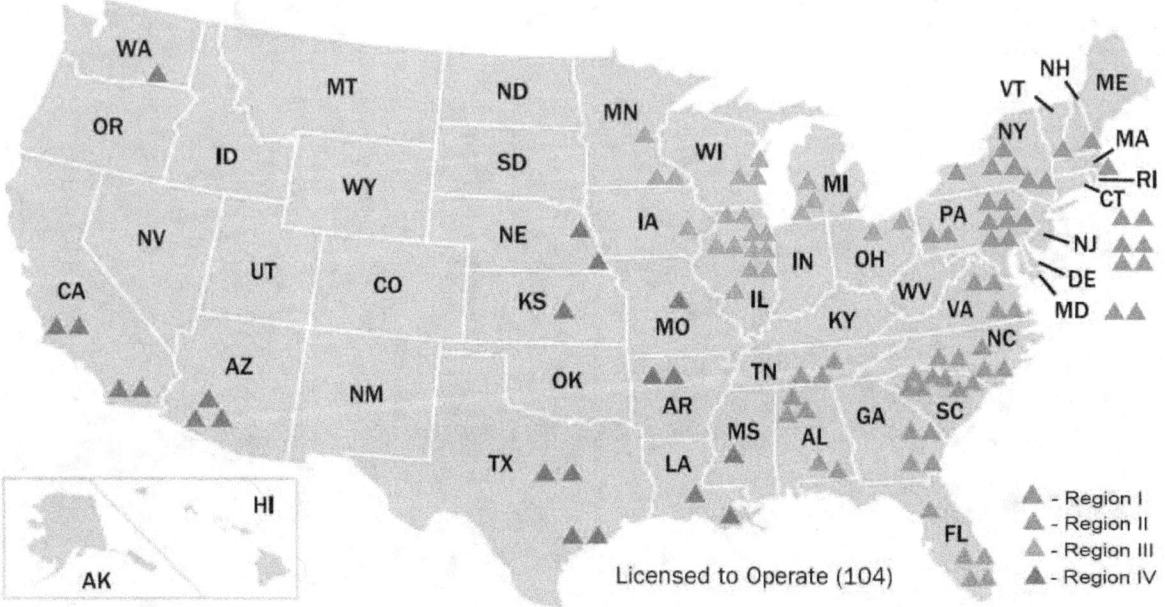

Licensed to Operate (104)

▲ - Region I
▲ - Region II
▲ - Region III
▲ - Region IV

THE LICENSE RENEWAL PROCESS

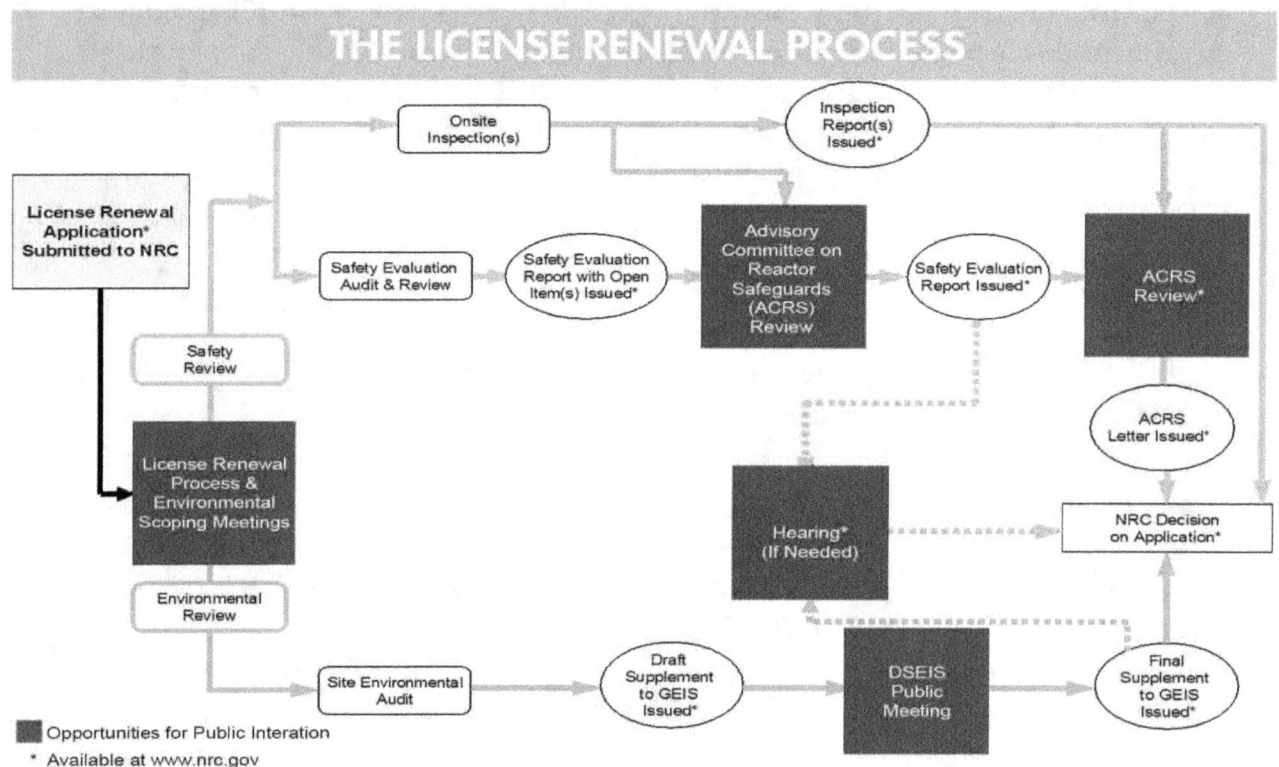

Opportunities for Public Interation

* Available at www.nrc.gov

The above flowchart illustrates the safety and environmental review process and the interrelationships among inspections, the Advisory Committee on Reactor Safeguards (ACRS) review, and the hearing process.

THE LICENSE RENEWAL PROCESS

The NRC license renewal process is effective and well established. Experienced NRC staff members conduct an extensive application review using well-defined schedules and communicate with all interested parties to actively involve the public in the license renewal process.

The environmental review and the safety review are the two components of reactor license renewal. The process for both reviews, which occur at the same time, generally takes between 22 and 30 months, depending on whether there is a hearing. Decisions to grant or deny a license renewal application are based on whether the applicant has demonstrated that it can meet the NRC's environmental and safety regulations during the period of extended operation.

ACRS conducts an independent safety review of license renewal applications and NRC staff evaluations. This independently appointedcommittee provides a forum where experts representing many technical perspectives give advice that is factored into the Commission's decision-making process. All license renewal ACRS meetings are open to the public and any member of the public may request an opportunity to make an oral statement during the committee meeting.

MORE INFORMATION

For more information on license renewal, including the status of current reviews, please visit the Reactor License Renewal Page at http://www.nrc.gov/reactors/operating/licensing/renewal.html.

THE SAFETY REVIEW

The NRC's top priority is ensuring that nuclear reactor facilities operate safely. The NRC performs a safety review of each license renewal application to be sure that the applicant has demonstrated that it will manage and monitor the effects of aging at the nuclear power facility during the period of extended operation.

In addition, inspectors travel to the nuclear power facility to verify the information in the renewal application and confirm that the aging management programs have been or are ready to be implemented. Following the safety review, the NRC prepares and makes available to the public a safety evaluation report.

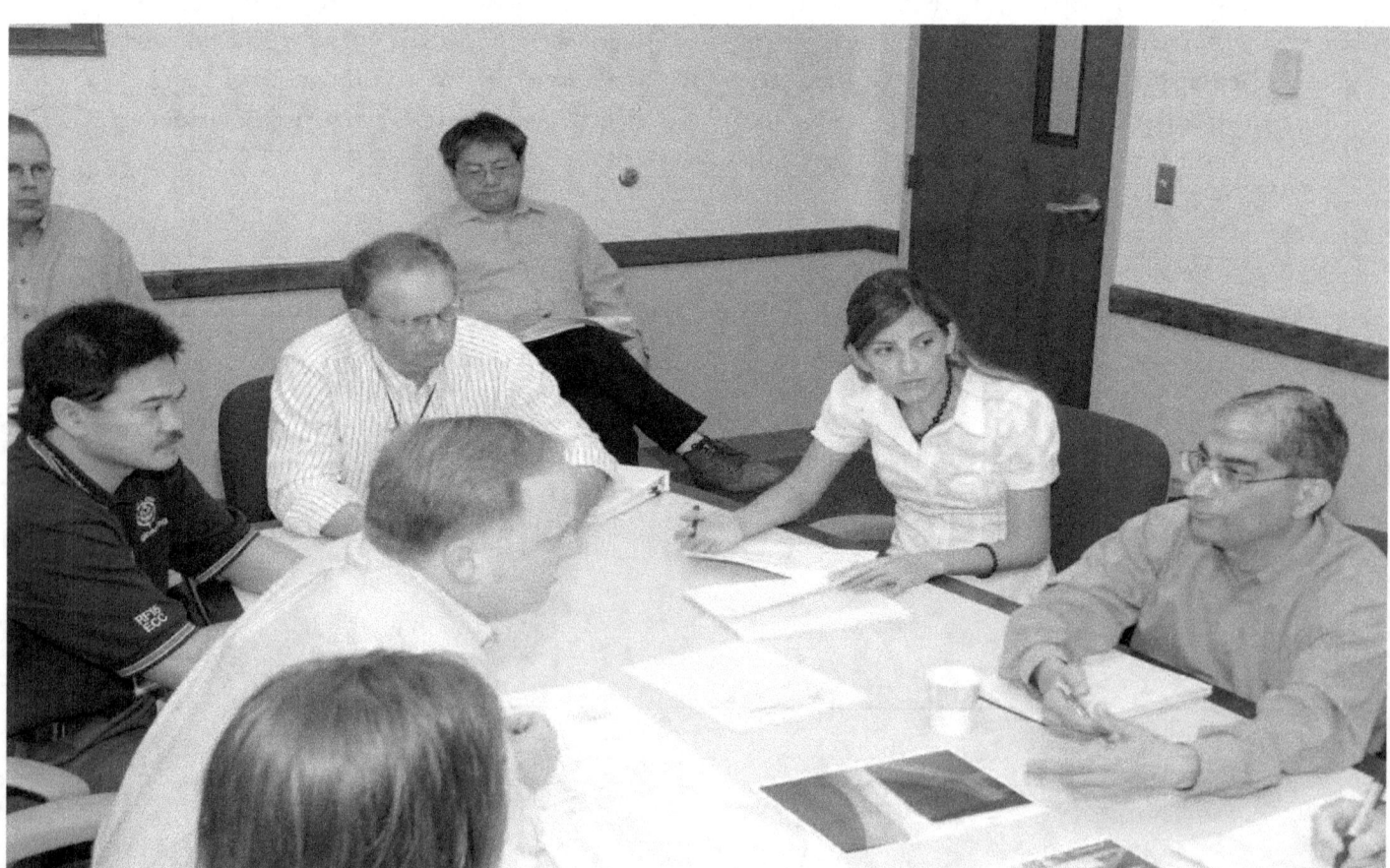

THE ENVIRONMENTAL REVIEW

The NRC also has responsibilities under the National Environmental Policy Act, which calls for a review of the environmental impact of reactor license renewal. Alongside its safety review, the NRC must investigate whether environmental issues related to the extension of the reactor's operating license exist.

The NRC has evaluated certain issues for all plants. NUREG-1437, "Generic Environmental Impact Statement for License Renewal of Plants" (GEIS), Volumes 1 and 2, May 1996, assessed the scope and impact of environmental effects that would be associated with license renewal at any nuclear power plant site.

A site-specific supplement to the GEIS is required for reactor license renewal. The NRC holds a "scoping" meeting near the plant to get input from the public and local officials on environmental issues they believe should be included in the supplement to the GEIS. The NRC then determines whether there are any environmental impacts that would affect license renewal.

The NRC publishes the draft supplement to the GEIS for public comment and holds public meetings. After consideration of comments on the draft, the NRC prepares and publishes a final supplement to the GEIS.

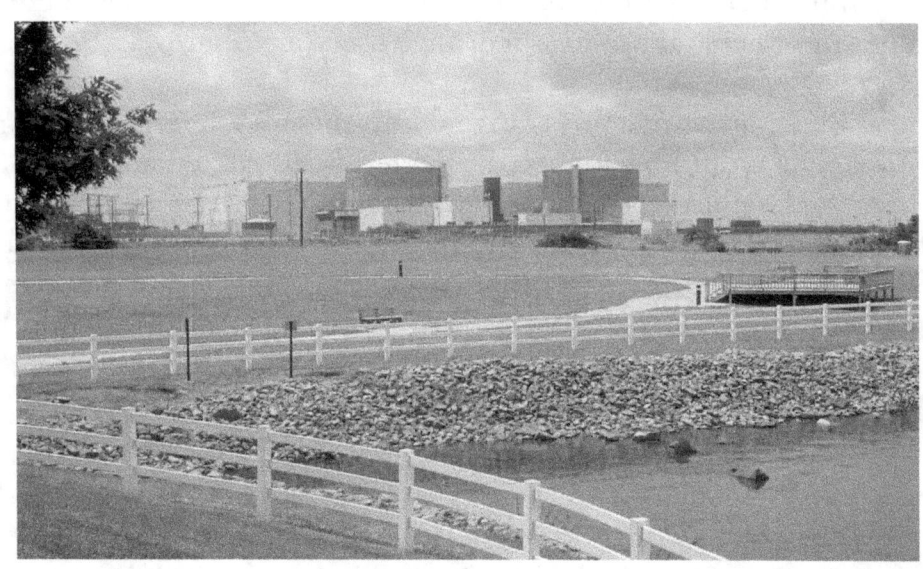

OPPORTUNITIES FOR PUBLIC INVOLVEMENT

Public participation is an important part of the license renewal process of a nuclear power facility. The typical license renewal process includes a number of meetings that are open to the public for the following purposes:

A meeting with the public to provide an overview of the license renewal process

A meeting with the public to discuss the scope of the environmental review and receive comments

A meeting with the public to discuss the draft site specific environmental impact statement and receive comments

Meetings with ACRS to discuss license renewal safety review

The NRC places notices in the *Federal Register* and local newspapers about upcoming public meetings. Meetings are also announced to the media via press releases and are listed on the NRC Web site under Public Meetings & Involvement. The NRC staff also notifies people who have previously attended public meetings related to a specific nuclear power facility or to license renewal in general about upcoming meetings that may be of interest.

Anyone can make a request for a formal adjudicatory hearing, or legal challenge, if he or she would be adversely affected by a particular license renewal. Anyone interested in filing for a hearing must submit a written request along with the contentions and supporting information. If the request for the hearing has proposed at least one contention that meets the requirements of the regulations, a hearing may be granted by the Atomic Safety and Licensing Board.

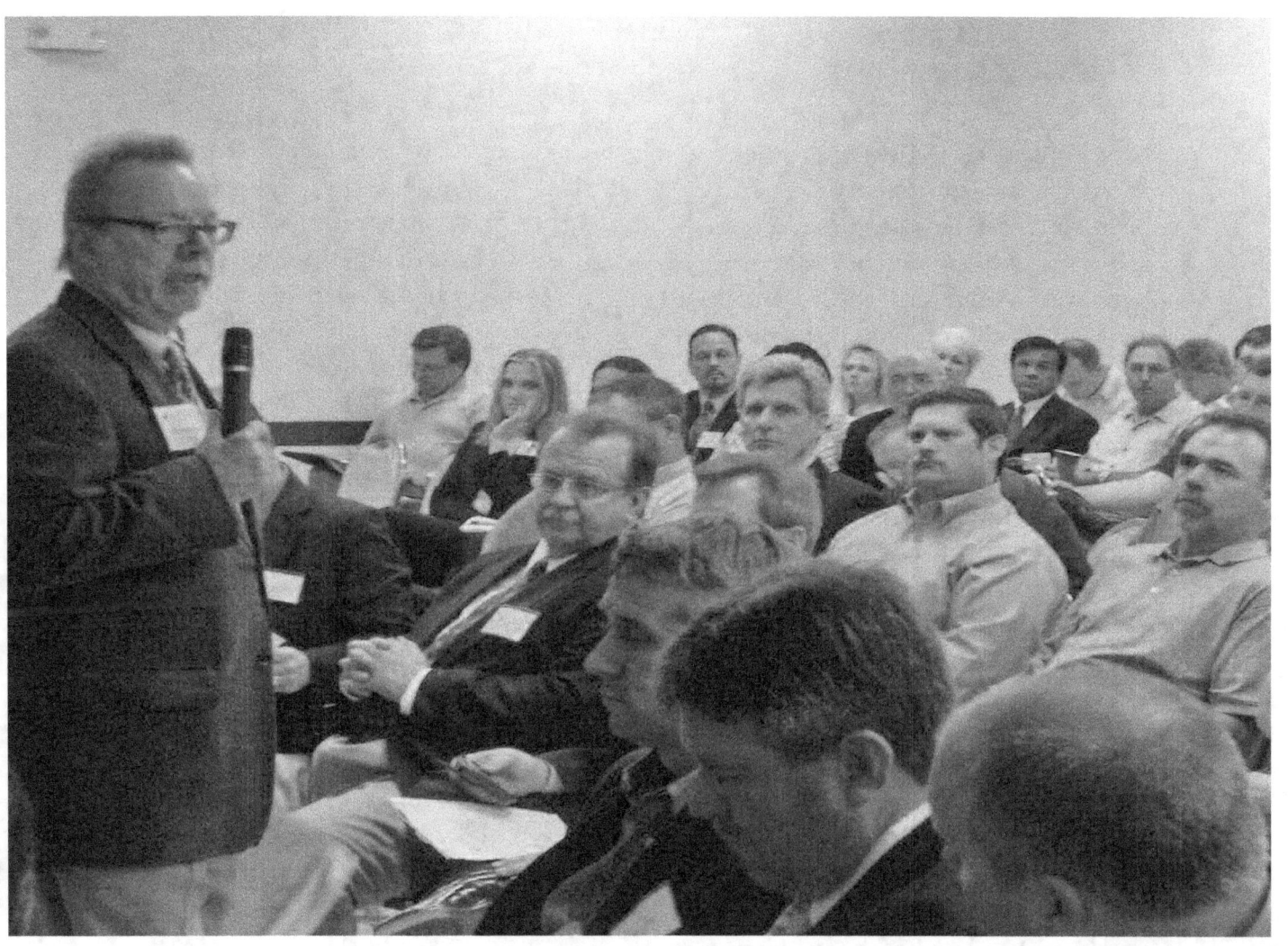

MORE INFORMATION

For more information on the hearing process, please visit the Reactor License Renewal Hearing Page (http://www.nrc.gov/reactors/operating/licensing/renewal/introduction/hearing.html.)

For more information on the hearing process, documents available for comment, and public meetings, please visit the Public Involvement in Reactor License Renewal Page (http://www.nrc.gov/reactors/operating/licensing/renewal/public involvement.html.)

WHICH REACTORS ARE UP FOR RENEWAL?

Forty percent of the existing nuclear reactor facilities have successfully completed the license renewal process. The owners of these facilities have demonstrated their understanding of the effects of aging on critical safety components and they have taken actions to ensure safe operation and minimal environmental impact during the period of extended operation.

About a third of the remaining 40-year reactor licenses will expire by the end of 2020. The total generating capacity of these nuclear power facilities would meet the electric needs of the entire population of the State of New York.

A nuclear power plant licensee may apply to the NRC to renew its license as early as 20 years before expiration of its current license. There is no limit on how late a licensee may apply for license renewal. However, if the licensee submits a renewal application that is sufficient for the NRC's review at least 5 years before expiration of its current license and the agency is still reviewing the application at the end of the 5 years, the plant can continue to operate until the NRC completes its review.

The list of approved license renewal applications, anticipated license renewal applications, and the status of pending applications can be obtained from the NRC Office of Public Affairs or on the NRC Web site (http://www.nrc.gov/reactors/operating/licensing/renewal/applications.html).

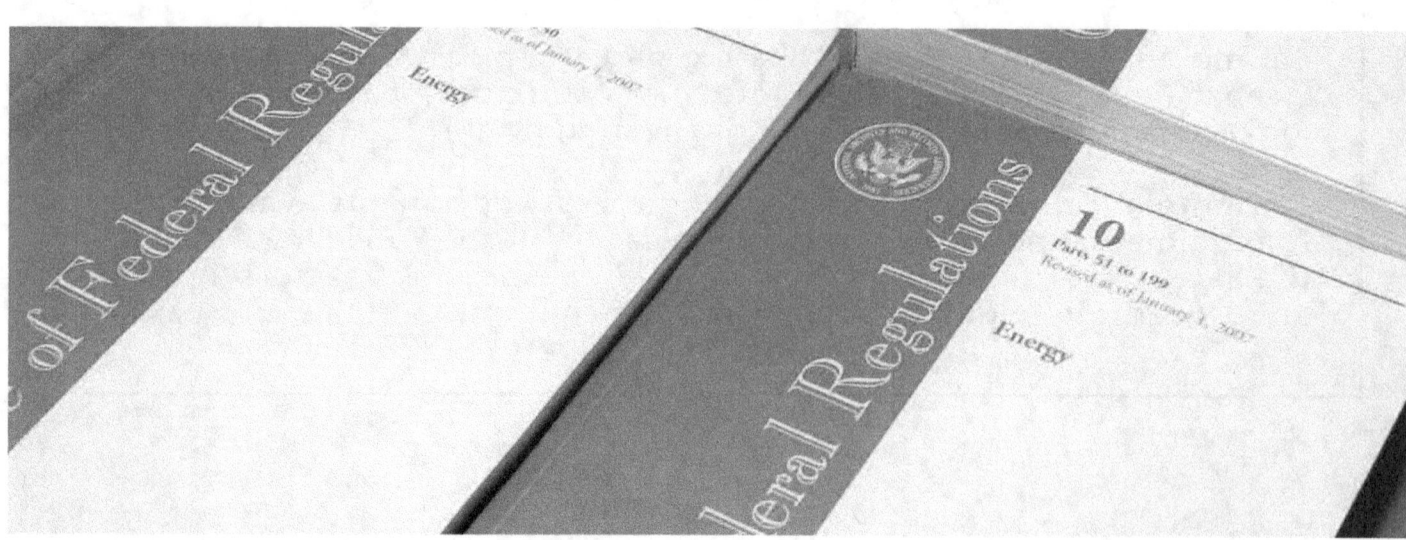

OPERATING NUCLEAR REACTORS

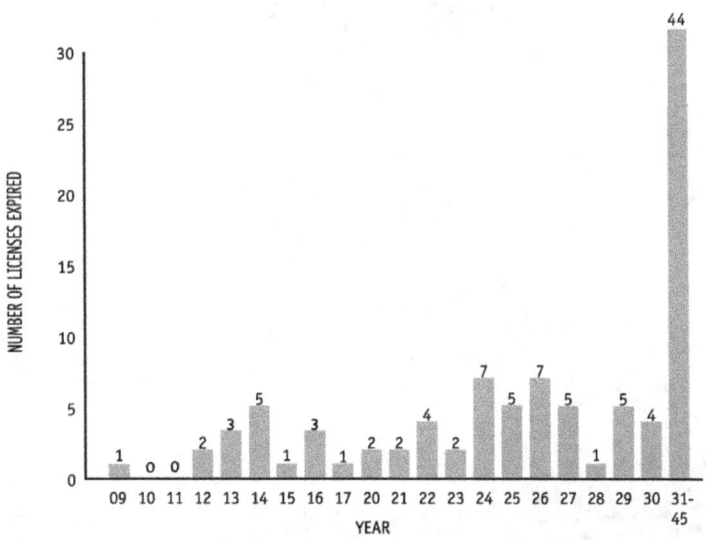

U.S. Commercial Nuclear Power Reactor Operating Licenses Expiration Date by Year, 2009–2046

2009	Oyster Creek
2012	Pilgrim 1
	Vermont Yankee
2013	Indian Point 2
	Kewaunee
	Prairie Island 1
2014	Cooper
	Duane Arnold
	James A. FitzPatrick
	Prairie Island 2
	Three Mile Island 1
2015	Indian Point 3
2016	Beaver Valley 1
	Crystal River 3
	Salem 1
2017	Davis-Besse
2020	Salem 2
	Sequoyah 1
2021	Diablo Canyon 1
	Sequoyah 2
2022	La Salle County 1
	San Onofre 2
	San Onofre 3
	Susquehanna 1
2023	La Salle County 2
	Columbia Generating St.

2024	Byron 1
	Callaway
	Grand Gulf 1
	Limerick 1
	Palo Verde 1
	Susquehanna 2
	Waterford 3
2025	Diablo Canyon 2
	Fermi 2
	Palo Verde 2
	River Bend 1
	Wolf Creek 1
2026	Braidwood 1
	Byron 2
	Clinton
	Hope Creek 1
	Perry 1
	Seabrook 1
	Shearon Harris 1
2027	Beaver Valley 2
	Braidwood 2
	Palo Verde 3
	South Texas Project 1
	Vogtle 1
2028	South Texas Project 2
2029	Limerick 2
	Dresden 2
	Ginna
	Vogtle 2
	Nine Mile Point 1

2030	Comanche Peak 1
	Robinson 2
	Point Beach 1
	Monticello
2031	Dresden 3
	Palisades
2032	Turkey Point 3
	Surry 1
	Quad Cities 1
	Quad Cities 2
2033	Browns Ferry 1
	Comanche Peak 2
	Fort Calhoun
	Oconee 1
	Oconee 2
	Peach Bottom 2
	Point Beach 2
	Turkey Point 4
	Surry 2
2034	Arkansas Nuclear 1
	Browns Ferry 2
	Brunswick 2
	Calvert Cliffs 1
	D.C. Cook 1
	Edwin Hatch 1
	Oconee 3
	Peach Bottom 3
2035	Watts Bar
	Millstone 2

2036	Browns Ferry 3
	Brunswick 1
	Calvert Cliffs 2
	St. Lucie 1
2037	Joseph M. Farley 1
	D.C. Cook 2
2038	Arkansas Nuclear 2
	Edwin Hatch 2
	North Anna 2
2040	North Anna 2
2041	Joseph M. Farley 2
	McGuire 1
2042	Summer
2043	Catawba 1
	Catawba 2
	McGuire 2
	St. Lucie 2
2045	Millstone 3
2046	Nine Mile Point 2

Note: Limited to reactors licensed to operate.

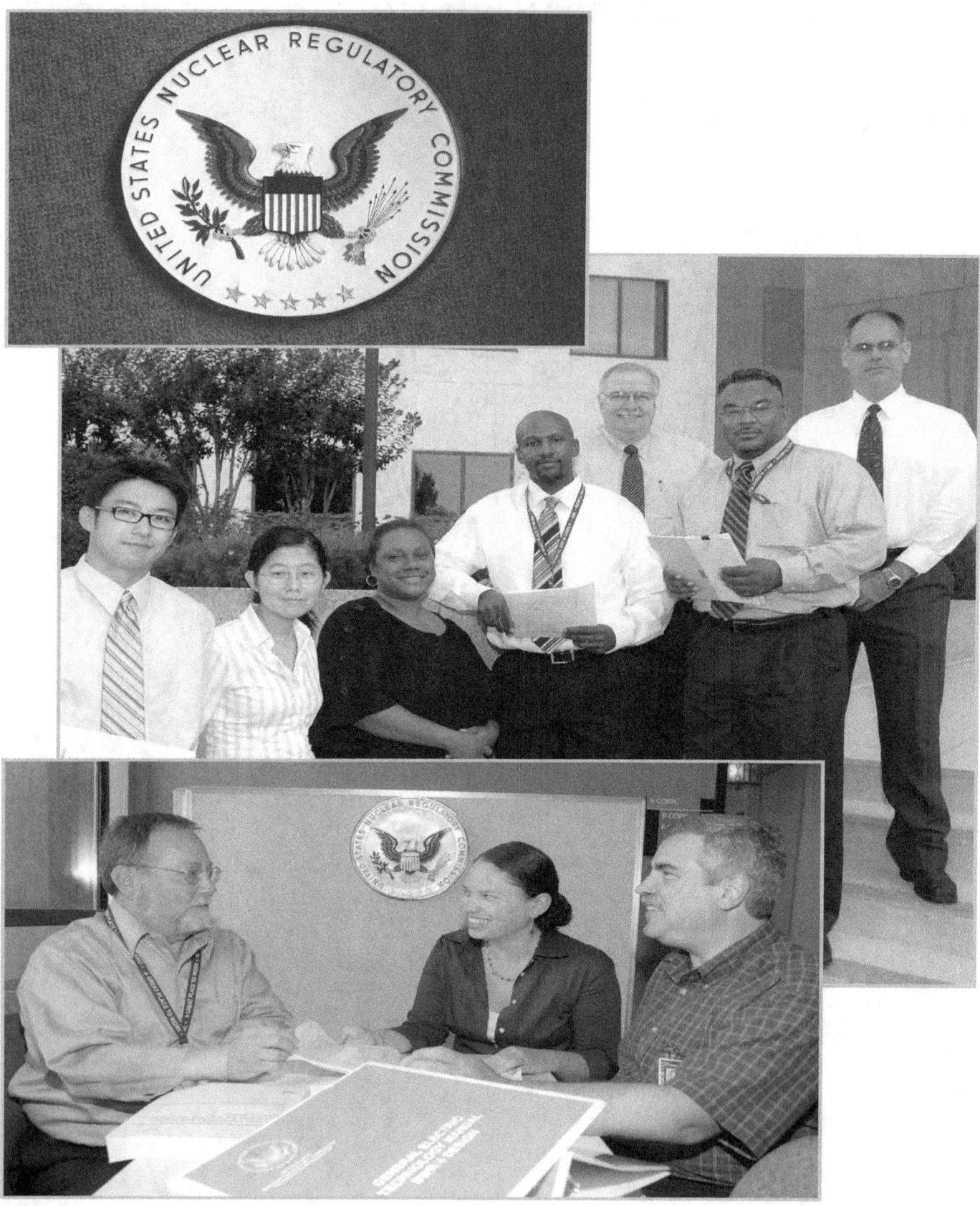

BRIAN HOLIAN

Division Director of License Renewal

As division director, Brian oversees all license renewal activities. His 18 years of experience at the NRC has included licensing activities, work at the Commission level, and nine years in Region I. He has a B.S. from Miami University in preengineering physics and an M.S. from the University of Southern California in systems management and was a former senior reactor operator in the industry.

"The process encourages participation. Many people are skeptical about nuclear power, while others see nuclear energy as a solution.   None of this affects our work; we do our work knowing that public safety is of utmost importance."

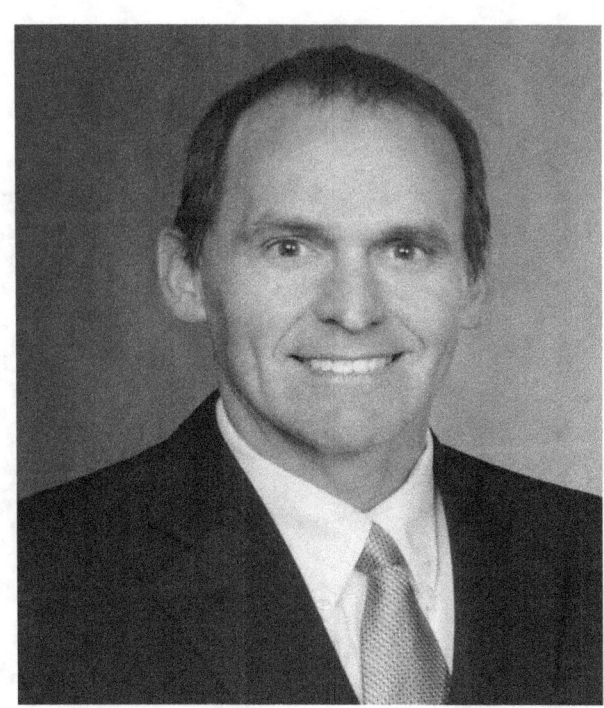

SAMSON LEE

Deputy Division Director

As deputy director of the license renewal division, Sam holds a key position at the NRC. He has a Ph.D. from MIT in mechanical engineering and has been with the agency for 20 years.

"The NRC's overriding task is to protect both the safety of the people and the environment. We have an amazing group dynamic where we make it a priority to work well together and help each other out, ensuring that we can go about the business of plant safety and protecting the environment."

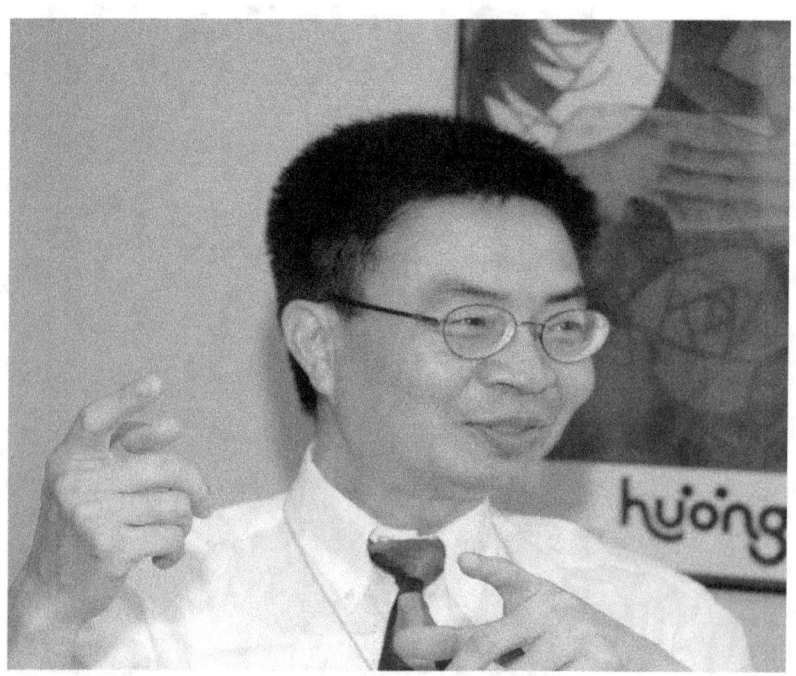

LOUISE LUND

Branch Chief

Louise oversees one branch of the license renewal division's safety reviewers, which focuses on the safety reviews for plants that seek 20-year extensions to their operating license. She has a B.S. as well as an M.S. in material sciences and engineering from Washington State University.

"The product we produce is our evaluation of a plant. It is the culmination of the work of many people who have applied their expertise in performing a technical review and reaching a common conclusion. Successful completion of the review process ensures that the plant can safely manage its aging for the next 20 years of operation."

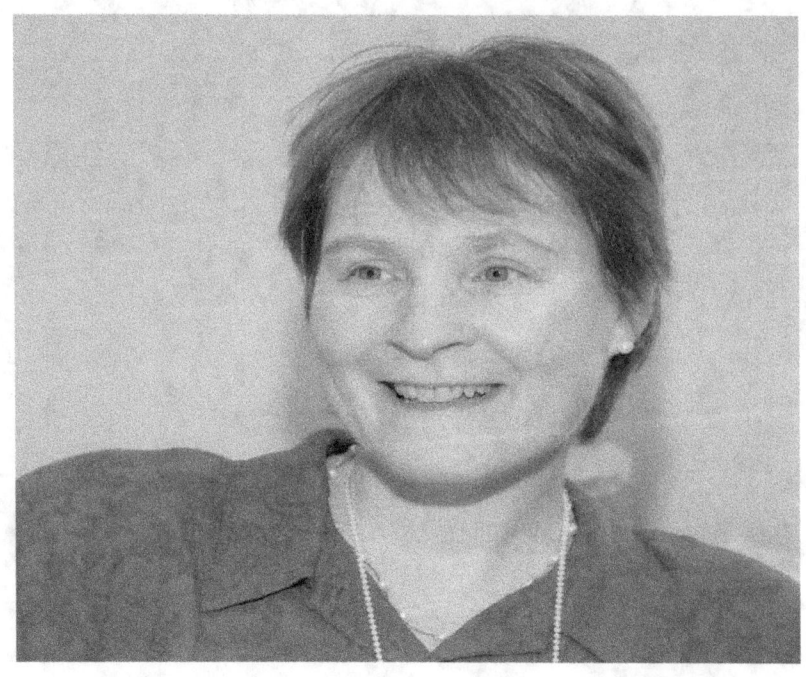

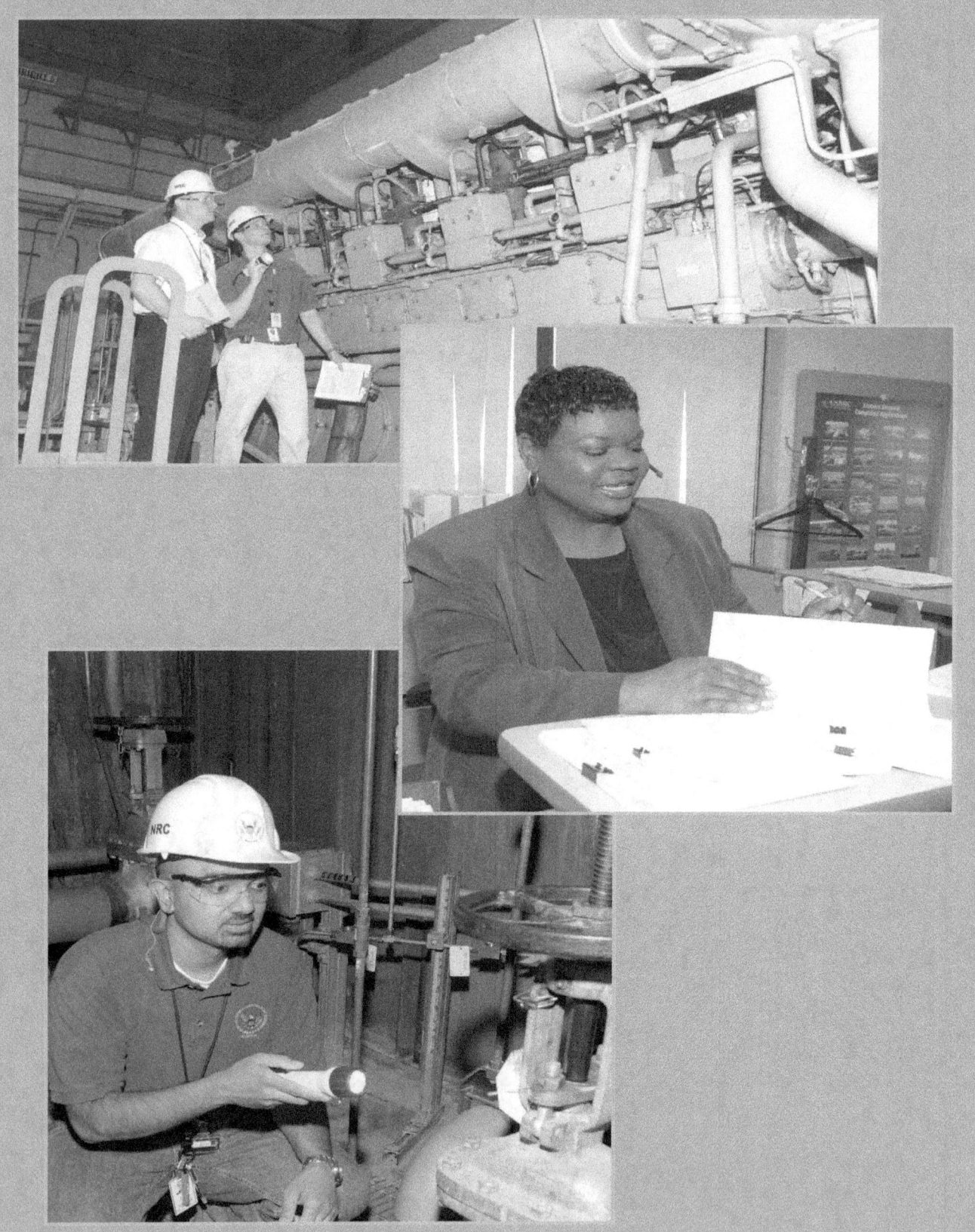

JEFFERY RIKHOFF

Senior Environmental Scientist

Jeffery has 20 years of experience in preparing environmental impact statements and environmental assessments. Currently, he oversees health physicists, biologists, hydrologists, archeologists, and economists who conduct the environmental review for all license renewal requests. He holds an M.S. in development economics and an M.R.P. in regional planning from the University of Pennsylvania.

"We have a wide range of environmental science experts who perform a rigorous review to determine the environmental impacts of operating a plant for an additional 20 years. This includes looking at the impacts on air, water, plants, and animals, as well as people. We perform this review in a very open manner, seeking public comments and consulting with other Federal, State and local organizations with environmental expertise. "

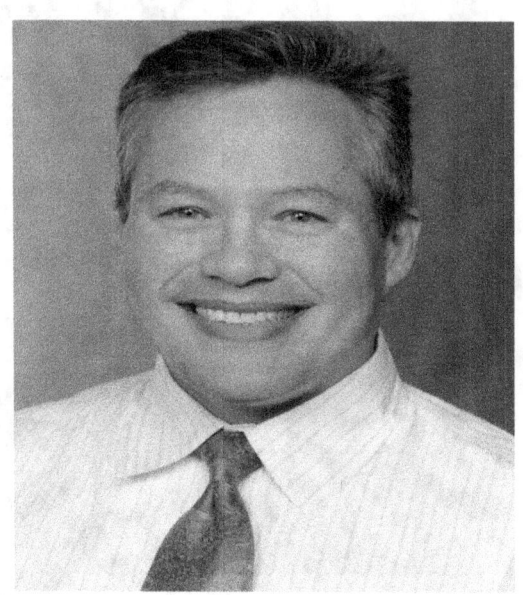

JIM MEDOFF

Senior Mechanical Engineer

Jim is a senior mechanical engineer who has been at the NRC for 18 years. He has an M.S. in material engineering from Drexel University.

"In looking to renew a license, we examine each infra-structure seam or line of tension with safety in mind to ensure that the plant will operate safely over the next 20 years."

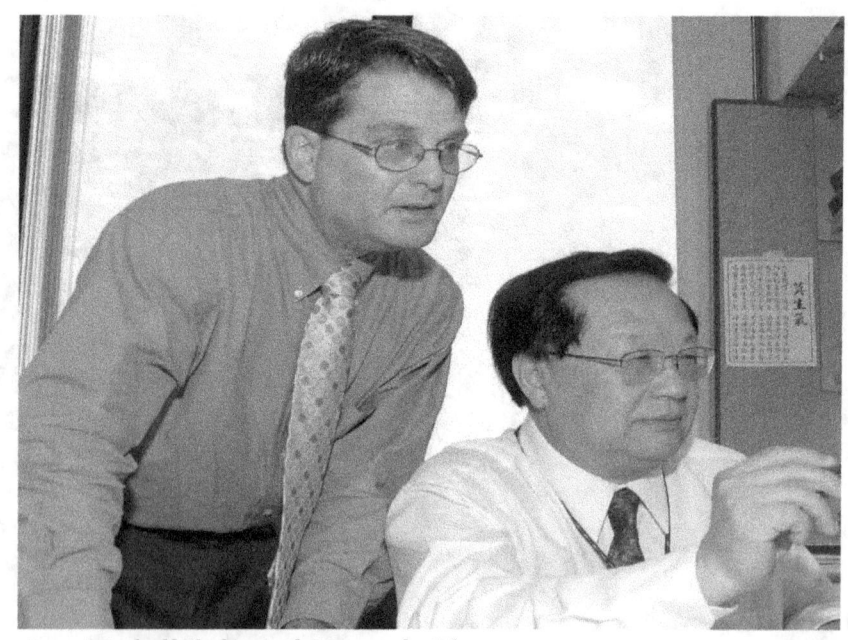

Jim Medoff (left) and Kenneth Chang

SAMUEL HERNANDEZ

Project Manager

Sam works at the NRC as an environmental programmer. He has a B.S. degree in chemical engineering from the University of Puerto Rico and a Master of Engineering in environmental engineering from the University of Maryland.

"I always thought someone was looking out for the public interests on issues of nuclear power. Now I realize I'm that person, and I take that responsibility very seriously. The NRC not only seeks out all points of view from the public on environmental issues, it also seeks all points of view from a diverse team of environmental professionals to ensure protection of the environment for the extended life of the plant."

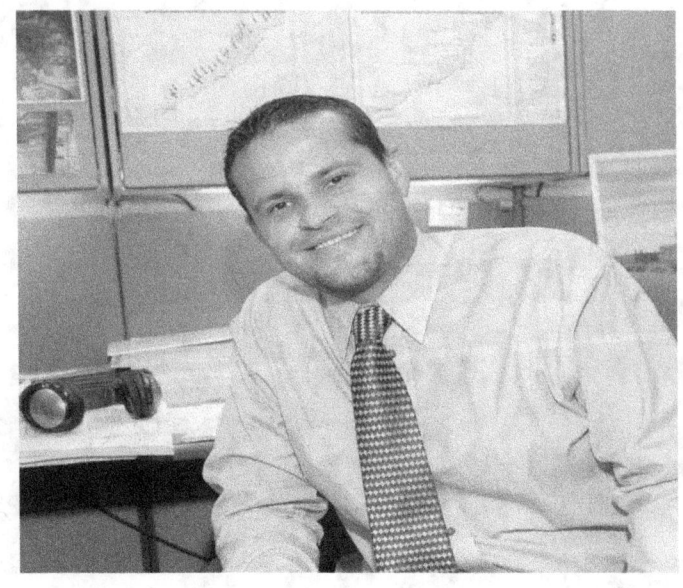

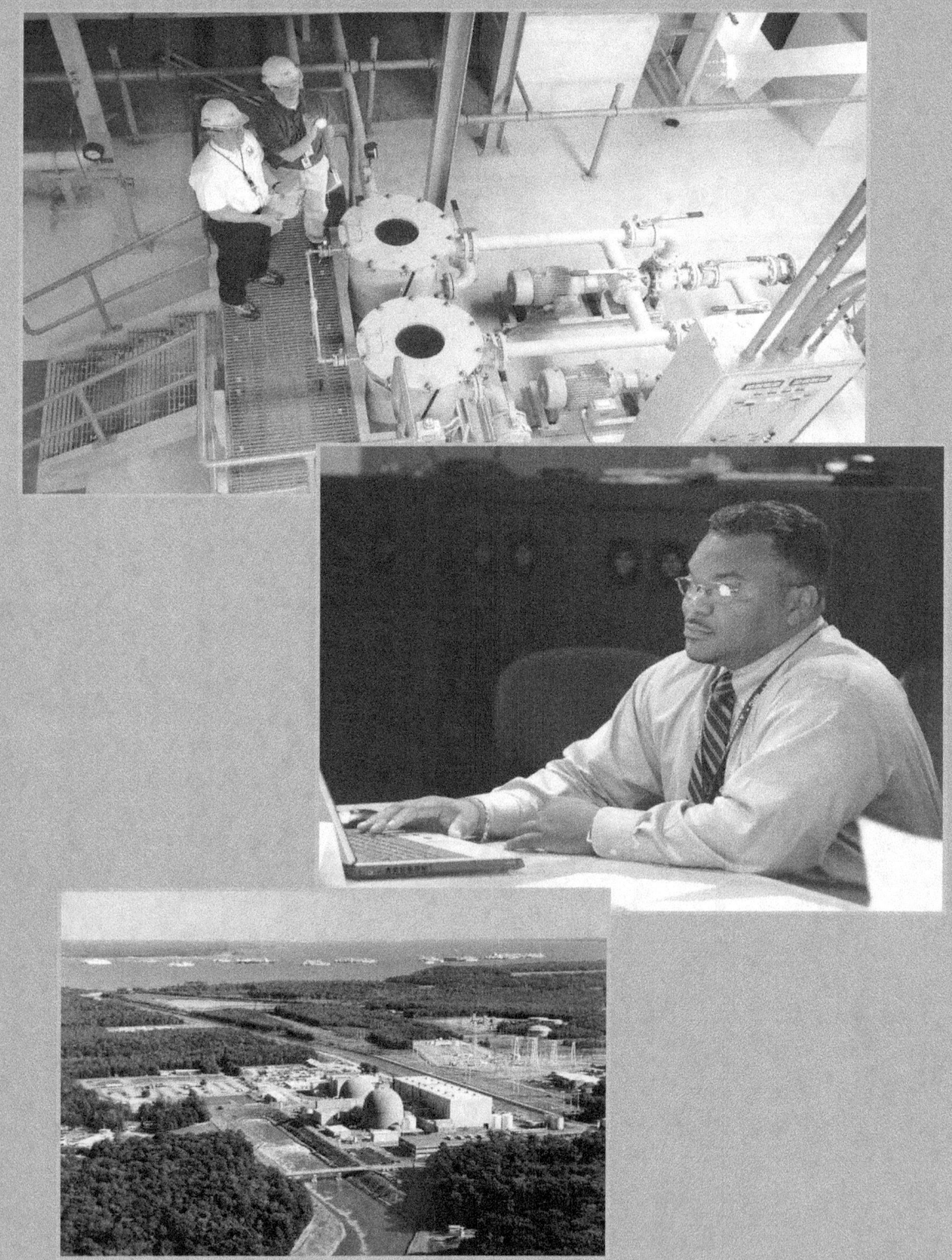

MAURICE HEATH

Project Manager

Maurice is a general engineer in the license renewal branch of the NRC. He has a B.S. degree in mechanical engineering from North Carolina Agricultural and Technical State University.

"We do a considerable amount of public outreach, and it is clear that many people have real concerns and want to be heard. Many are concerned with safety, and many are concerned about the jobs the plants bring. My goal is to make sure the public understands the relicensing process so they can participate. Public health and safety is our top priority."

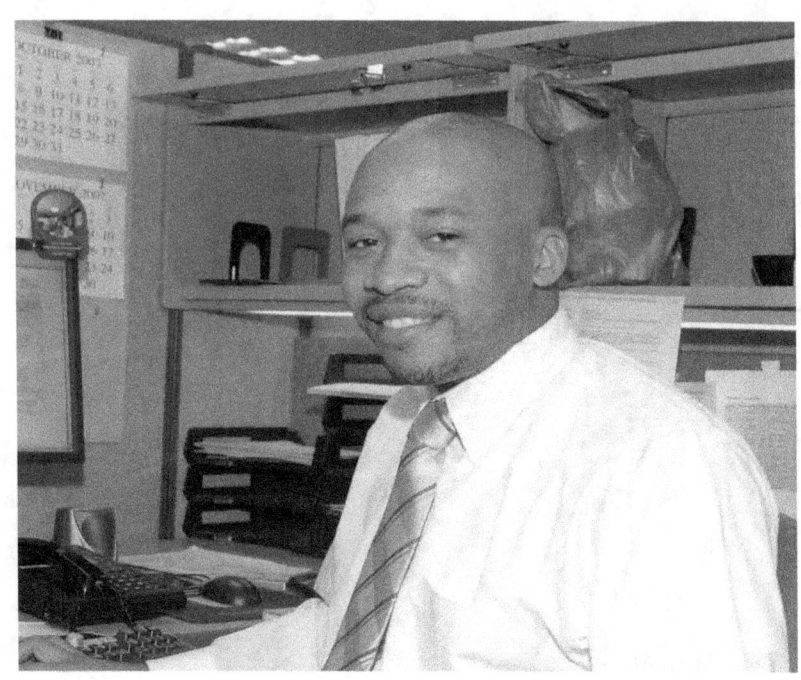

JIM DAVIS

Senior Materials Engineer

Jim has 18 years of experience working as a materials engineer in the nuclear industry. He received his B.S., M.S., and Ph.D. in metallurgical engineering from Ohio State.

"The bottom line is that we make sure everything in a plant is safe and will remain safe."

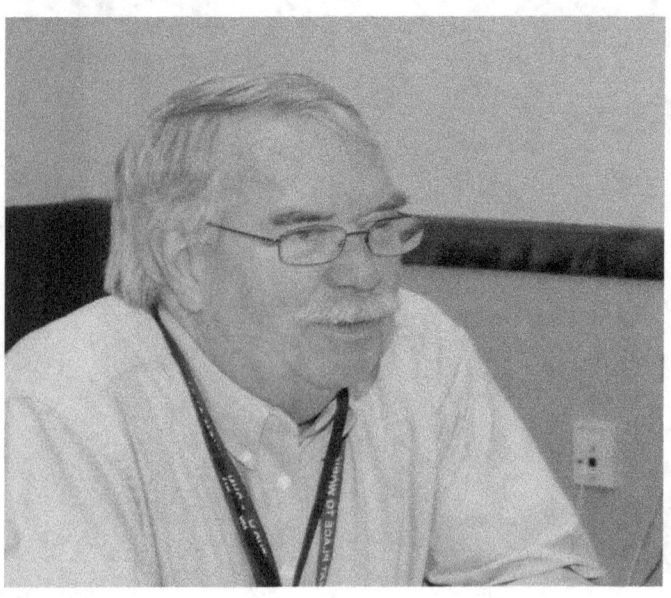

STEVE KLEMENTOWICZ

Senior Health Physicist

Steve has been a senior health physicist for the NRC for more than 17 years. He has an M.S. in health physics from the University of Florida.

"We all take the responsibility of public trust seriously. I was trained in health physics. We all understand there is no room for bias in the rules and regulations of the NRC. We conduct our inspections with complete objectivity. It is an awesome responsibility."

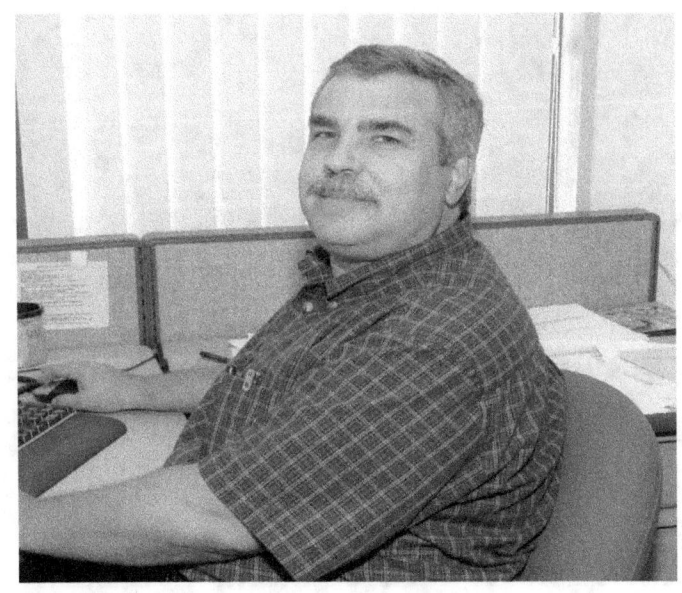

JONATHAN ROWLEY

Project Manager

Jonathan is a lead project manager for the NRC's safety review of a given license renewal application and coordinates the NRC's safety evaluation report of that license renewal application. He earned an M.S. in materials engineering from the University of Texas at Arlington.

"We understand that there are people who feel unsure about nuclear power. In truth, some of the smartest men and women work at the NRC. While they understand these reservations, they know the expert level of knowledge that has been applied in the review process and all are committed to ensuring the safety of the community."

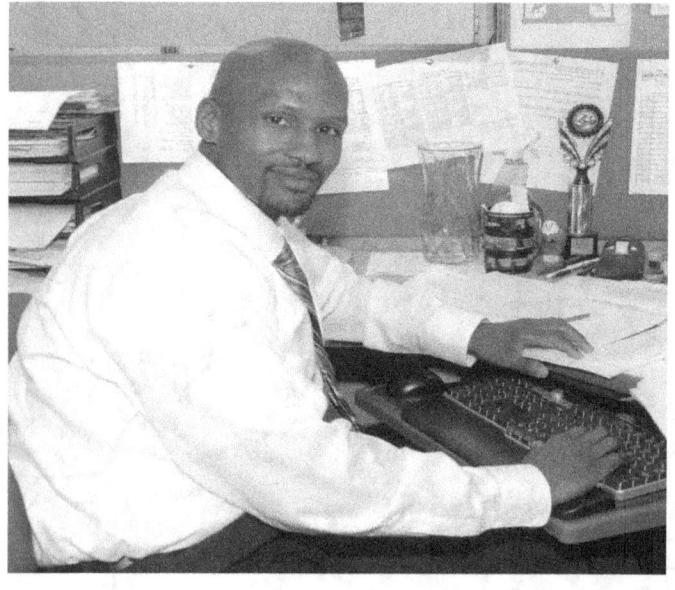

VERONICA RODRIGUEZ

Project Manager

Veronica has worked for the NRC for 5 years, first as a reactor engineer before taking on her current responsibilities as lead project manager. Veronica earned a B.S. in chemical engineering from the University of Puerto Rico and a master's degree in project management from the University of Maryland.

"The ongoing health and safety of the public are paramount to the NRC, as is providing the public access to information about the license renewal process. We take very seriously our responsibility to protect the public and the environment and are committed to providing opportunities for the public to participate in the license renewal process and have their questions and concerns addressed in a timely manner."

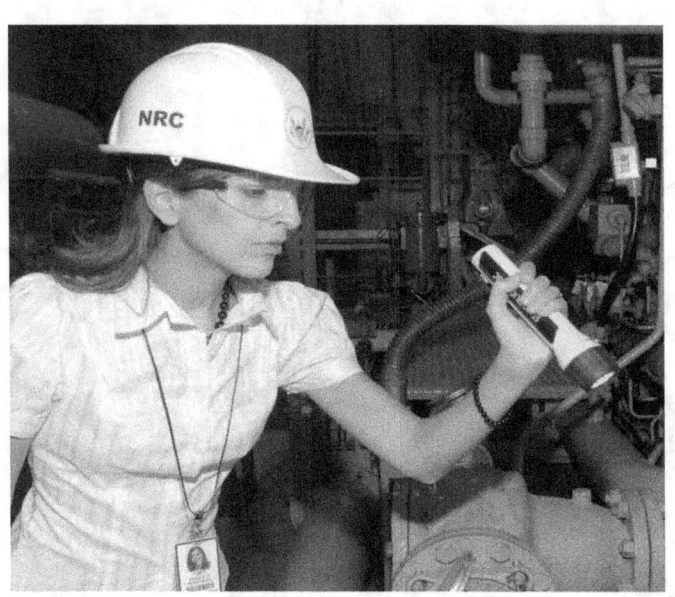

For the past 20 years, the NRC has been studying and refining the license renewal process.

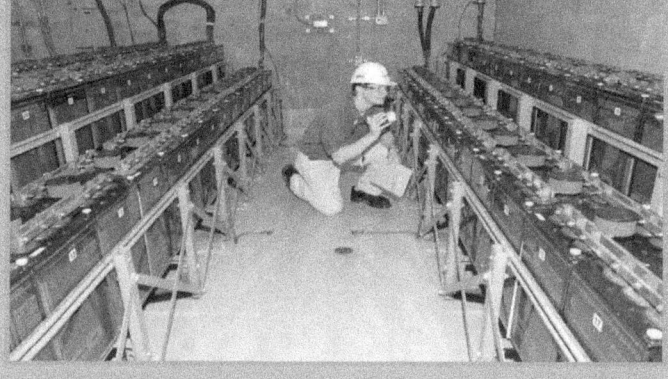

The NRC's top priority is ensuring nuclear reactor facilities operate safely.

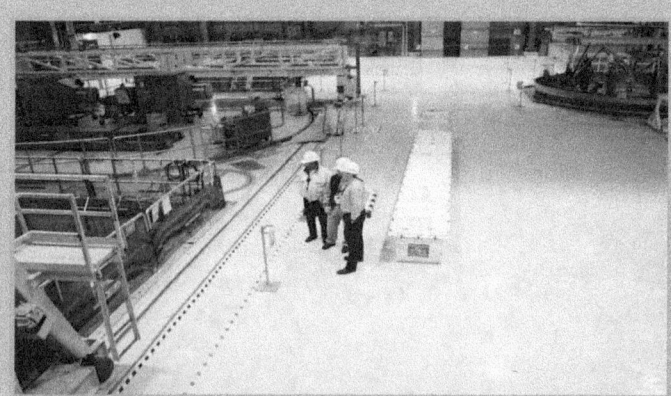

ACRS conducts an independent safety review of license renewal applications and NRC staff evaluations. This independently appointed committee provides a forum where experts representing many technical perspectives provide advice that is factored into the Commission's decision-making process.

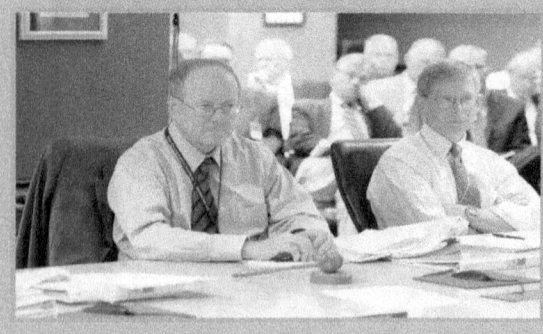

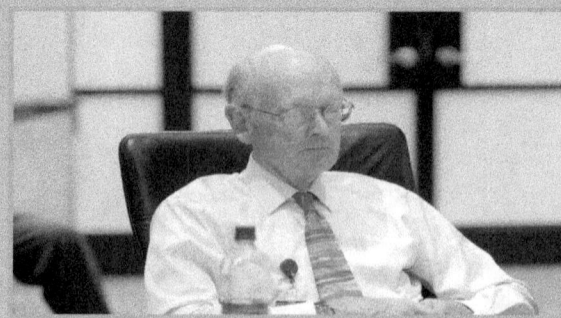

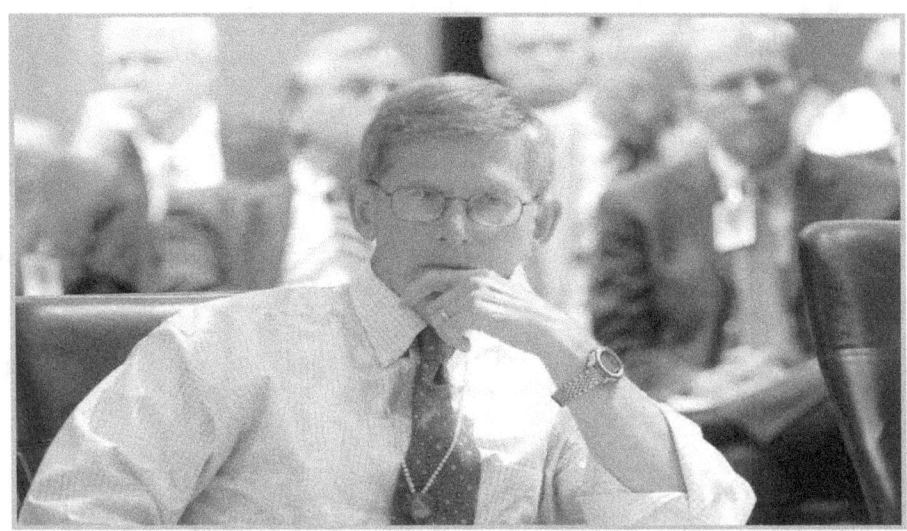

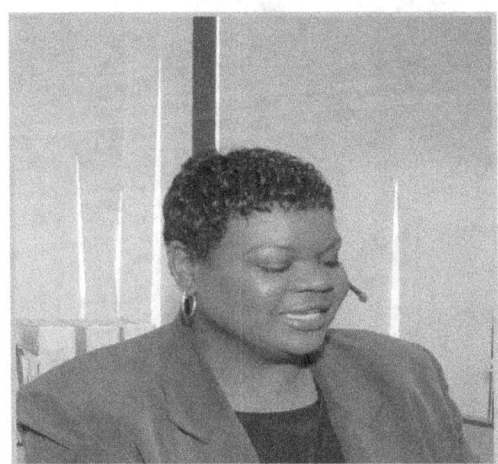

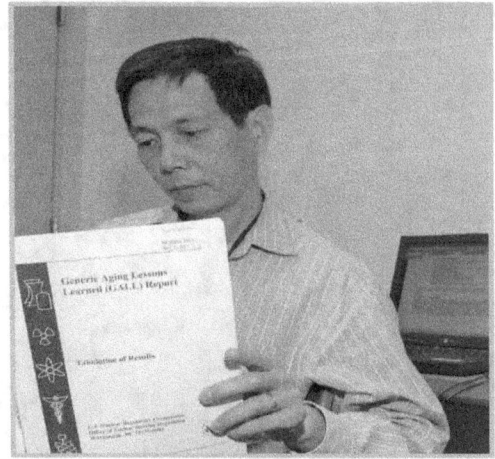

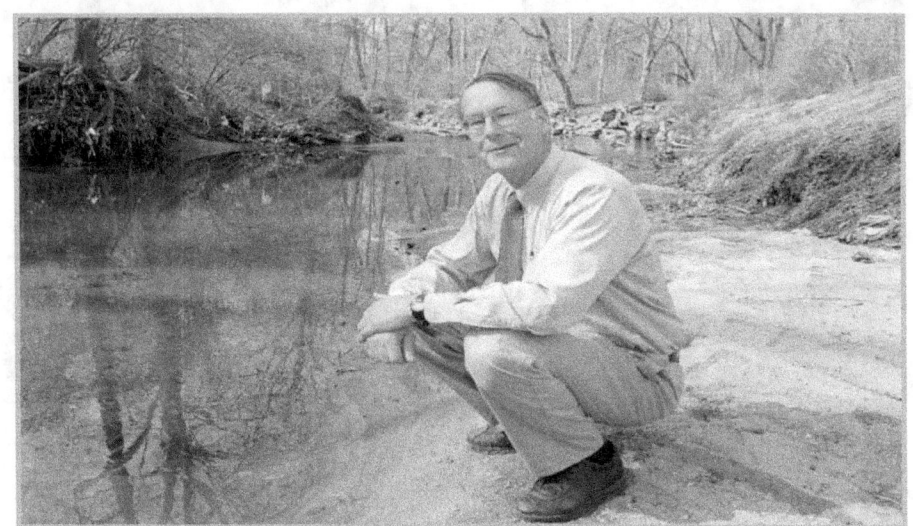

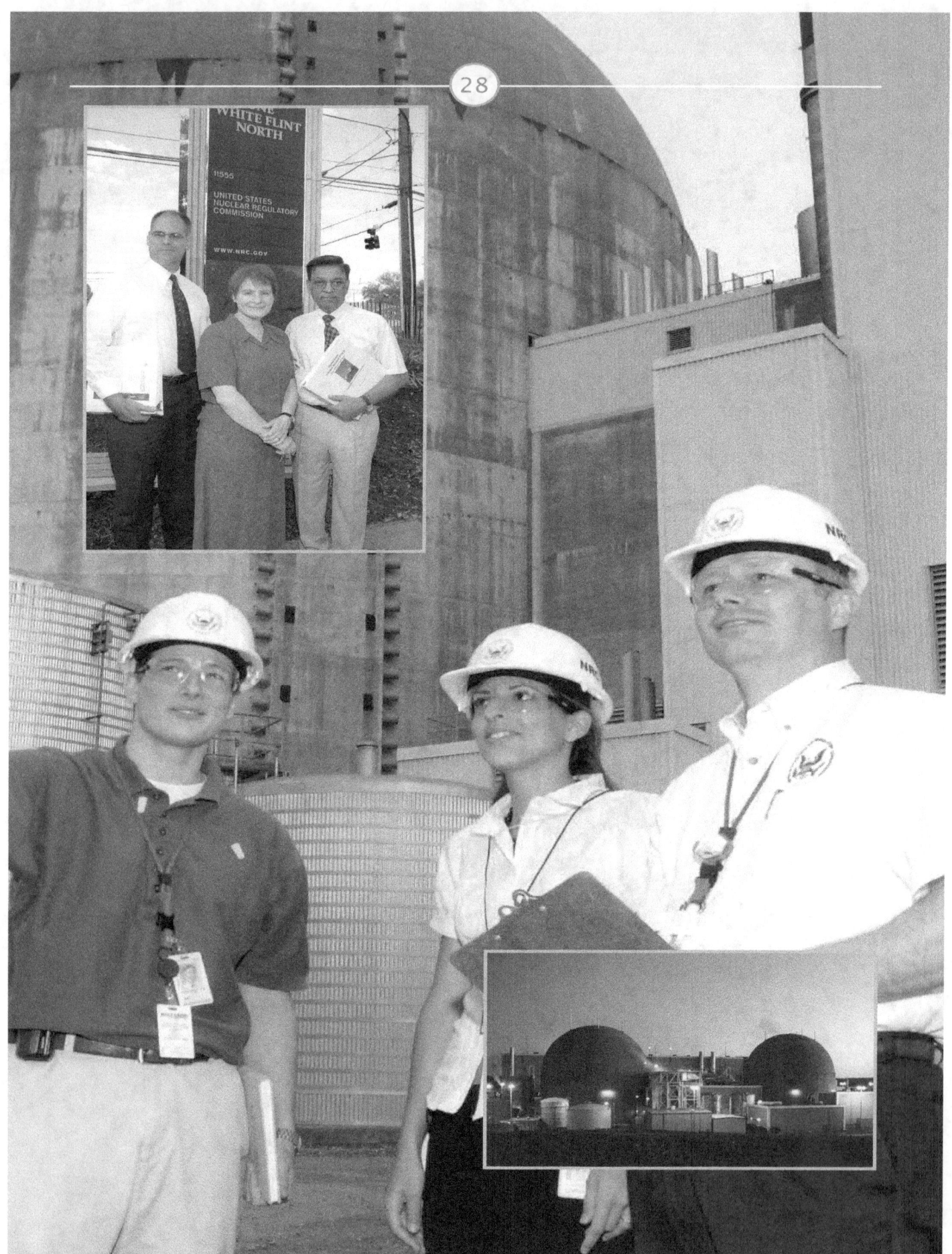

MORE INFORMATION

Reactor License Renewal Page
(http://www.nrc.gov/reactors/operating/licensing/renewal.html.)

Reactor License Renewal Introduction Page (http://www.nrc.gov/
reactors/operating/licensing/renewal/introduction/hearing.html.)

Public Involvement in Reactor License Renewal Page
(http://www.nrc.gov/reactors/operating/licensing/renewal/
public involvement.html.)

Office of Public Affairs
U.S. Nuclear Regulatory Commission
Washington, DC 20555 0001

Telephone: (301) 415 8200
or (800) 368 5642
Fax: (301) 415 2234

Email: OPA@NRC.GOV

www.nrc.gov

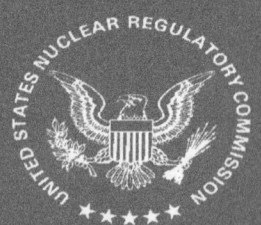

NUREG/BR-0291, Rev. 2
January 2009